Love-Song
Paul Laurence Dunbar

If Death should claim me for her own to-day,
And softly I should falter from your side,
Oh, tell me, loved one,
would my memory stay,
And would my image in your heart abide?
Or should I be as some forgotten dream,
That lives its little space, then fades entire?
Should Time send o'er you
its relentless stream,
To cool your heart, and quench for aye love's fire?

I would not for the world, love, give you pain,
Or ever compass what would
cause you grief;
And, oh, how well I know that tears are vain!
But love is sweet, my dear, and life is brief;
So if some day before you I should go
Beyond the sound and sight of
song and sea,
'T would give my spirit stronger wings to know
That you remembered still and wept for me.

Beyond the Pink Ribbon:

My Spiritual Journey through Breast Cancer

Rev. Dr. Rhonda Rhea

JS Publishing and Consulting, LLC
3401 12th Street, NE #29563
Washington, DC 20017
jspublishing.me
www.justsistersnetwork.org

Copyright, 2010, 2020
ISBN: 978-0-9795060-4-8
Library of Congress Control No:
2020921886

The West African Adinkra Symbol used
through this book means "By God's grace, all will be
well." It is a symbol for hope, providence and faith.

This book is dedicated
In Memory of Jan Lynn Clemons
and to all the other warriors
who pressed their way through.

For as long as I can remember, pink has always been my favorite color. I get a renewed energy every time I am in the presence of something pink. As October, Breast Cancer Awareness Month, comes around you see pink ribbons everywhere. We have all come to understand what it represents: both awareness and hope.

Whether it is a lapel pin or on the products you purchase, there is an all-out effort to bring awareness about the ills of breast cancer and a call to eradicate this disease in our lifetime.

On many fronts it is a war of sorts. There are groups advocating for more funding. There are groups advocating for more testing. Early detection seems to be the most dominate solution in this war on cancer. Yet through all of the information and outreach efforts, women are still dying at staggering rates. Oftentimes there are so many questions unanswered. What more can be done? Why is this happening to me? Will I survive this?

Yes, the pink ribbon has become both a symbol of hope as well as a badge of honor for survival. But breast cancer is not an isolated disease. It is truly a community disease because the impact is so profound. When you think about the women impacted by the disease of breast cancer, you must also include their family and friends. The amount of worry, stress, fear, and even the anguish that friends and family members feel is so vastly understated.

So, I find it ironic that my all-time favorite color pink would be connected to something that has completely changed and defined my life.

I am inspired to tell my story because it pierces the veil of the breast cancer experience. My story is like so many others who have survived this war and have come to experience life, beyond the pink ribbon.

Table of Contents

This is my story, this is my song...

Blessed Assurance

I am a survivor that much I know for sure. And this is my story. I was speaking with a friend on New Year's Day and I told her that I felt as if I had been through a car wash, with no car. As the darkness fell in my life, I was overtaken by the blinding and pouring water falling down. I felt the soapy brushes grinding out everything that I have known and loved. I endured the side to side pounding of the heavy wet rags. Could I take anymore? Just then, the intense heat showed up and everything dried. Finally, a little light emerges. And as I entered into the sunlight, I realized that the journey was so worth it because at the end of the ride, I was hand polished and dried off by the best-- God himself.

I believe that everything is perfectly planned, coordinated and orchestrated by God. In the normal sequence of life, it is usually better to tell a story from the beginning but in my situation, the ending is the beginning because of how God's hand has moved in my life.

I was diagnosed with Stage II breast cancer on May 1, 2003. On May 25, 2006, I was told that the cancer had aggressed to Stage IV and that there was no hope and no possibility of surviving. I lived with "active cancer" since the date of my diagnosis. On May 1, 2010, I reached seven years of living with cancer. From a spiritual perspective seven is God's number for completion. On June 1, 2010, I learned that I am now cancer-free.

Yes, I have a story to tell you. It is rooted in an unwavering faith. What is so extraordinary about my experience is that it has truly been a modern-day journey of biblical proportions. I have been like Job, or as a friend of mine often refers to me as Jobette. I know fire and I know rain. I know famine and I know lack. I know affliction and I know despair. But even as these things appeared in my life, I always trusted God. I never wavered on my faith. I trusted God's miraculous, healing power. Even though I was spiritually young, so to speak, I knew with certainty, that God, all by himself, was going to heal me and that I was going to survive. I had this knowing, even when others had their doubts.

But what I did not know was how much I would thrive. Because through this journey, I grew to know God on a whole other level that is difficult to explain except to say, that I am in the best space in my life. I have a freedom and a total dependency on God that I would not have otherwise known.

I am writing this book to share my story in hopes that it will inspire other warriors to press on. Having breast cancer is truly not the worst thing that could happen in my life. I will admit that it was a challenge. But more than that, breast cancer actually served as a liberator. I FEAR **NOTHING** and I TRUST GOD for *EVERYTHING*.

I made a promise to God that when I was able to speak about this aspect of my life, I would entitle it, "Coming to My Spiritual Senses". In July of 2008, at the urging of many friends, I gave my first speech with that title. It now serves as the basis of this book.

As I have learned through this spiritual journey, there is nothing greater than God's love. I am most appreciative that God found me worthy to be the vessel to bring this story to you. Because in knowing my story, you too will know that it really is all about God.

As the darkness fell

Dear brothers and sisters, when troubles come
your way, consider it an opportunity for great joy.
For you know that when your faith is tested,
your endurance has a chance to grow.
So let it grow,
for when your endurance is fully developed,
you will be perfect and complete,
needing nothing.
James 1:2-4
New Living Translation

The Gentle Pull

My breast cancer journey actually began with an embrace. I was on vacation in Jamaica in July of 2002 and in a single act of tenderness; just like the gentle tug at the beginning of a car wash, this journey began.

As my dear friend Leroy greeted me with a hug, he immediately pushed me away. The tumor in my left breast was so profound that it could be felt in a hug. Leroy asked me if I was aware of the now obvious tumor in my breast. And immediately, I defended the tumor. Like many African American women, I was diagnosed with fibrocystic breast. The benign tumor, that was now in question, had been in my breast since 1984.

In 1996, doctors discovered two additional tumors in the left breast, and they were immediately removed. The original tumor, however, was not removed. The surgeon reasoned that since it had been there for such a long time and since it was not causing a problem, that it would be best, just to leave it alone. So, with this new discovery on this warm July afternoon, I felt no urgency about "that" tumor.

My friend Leroy, however, was very concerned as he asked me to "check about it" when I got back home. But I *KNEW* that there was nothing to worry about.

While I was still in Jamaica, I contacted Neeka, also a good friend. Because my hair had been thinning and balding, I asked Neeka to twist it for me. As Neeka was doing my hair, she suggested that I use some castor oil to help strengthen it.

I went the next day and I bought some castor oil from the drug store. I then contacted Neeka to let her know that I had purchased the castor oil. When Neeka stopped by, she immediately began to scold me in a gentle way.

She said, "Oh no Rhonda, this will not do. You must have pure castor oil, the kind they make in the mountains." She told me that she was going to have some castor oil made for me.

Two days later as I was pulling away to catch my flight, Neeka was literally running with this small container of castor oil in her hand. What struck me as odd was not just the fact that she was running, but how protectively she was carrying this bottle. Neeka had such an urgent and a determined look on her face, that it actually frightened me.

Neeka placed the bottle of castor in my hand. She expressed my need for the castor oil and that she would keep me in her prayers. It was as if she understood something very profound and she was lovingly trying to prepare me.

I returned home from Jamaica. My life at the time was very chaotic, very stressful, and very compressed. Time to do anything outside of my daily routine, was an all time premium.

I put the tumor on the bottom of my list of things to do and I went on with life as it came rushing towards me. My biggest health challenge at the time was the management of stroke-level hypertension. No matter what medication was prescribed, my body was non-responsive. The blood pressure continued to rise.

Each month, I performed my monthly breast examination. The tumor was in the exact location that it has always been and even though the tumor was very large, I had no sense that anything could possibly be wrong.

In the spring of 2003, I finally took the time to have a complete physical examination, including a mammogram. I did not think anymore about it. The tumor was massive, but I had begun to think that maybe, it had always been that large. I literally had no worry or no concern.

I got a call from my doctor's office on Tuesday, April 29, 2003 stating that they wanted to go over the report with me. I asked them to send it in the mail and they did.

♥ The Envelope, Please

I received the medical report in the mail on Thursday, May 1, 2003. I was at my then 91-year-old grandmother's house and it had been a very hectic day. My sister Monica was traveling out of town at the time and I had the sole responsibility of the family business: employees and payroll, students and parents. I was also responsible for my sister's daughter, Rhea and for my son, Carson. It was a big responsibility for any one person, on a regular day, but on this day, it was exceptionally stressful.

My instinct had directed me to the porch so that I could read the letter in privacy. Because of my history with fibroid tumors, the anticipated result of a mammogram was really, no big deal.

I opened the envelope and I took out the letter which was carefully folded in thirds. The first part of the letter confirmed my suspicion; the tumor that had been in my left breast for almost twenty years was calcified, just like I thought – nothing to worry about.

I opened the second part of the letter and froze as I read, "intraductal carcinoma – HIGHLY SUSICIOUS AS MALIGNANT. And then I opened the third fold and it revealed, METATISIS in the right lymph node.

Oh my God!

As I read that letter, fold after fold, I cannot explain to you the fear and the panic that came over me. I begin to break out in a sweat, my heart began to race fast. I felt that everything in my body was about to come right out of my mouth. My knees became weak and at any moment I felt as if I was going to hit the ground. Malignant – Metastasis, those words kept pound in my head.

Oh my God! This cannot be happening to me.

I picked up the telephone and called my girlfriend Jacque. We have been friends since we were in the Kindergarten. Her mother had died from breast cancer so I knew that she would understand the medical terms that were in the report. In her always calm voice, she said, "Rhonda, let's not panic, let's wait until all of the test are done." "PANIC," I yelled at her. "This report says that I am dead already and you say not to PANIC".

I must admit to you that I did not know what to do. I was in a real panic, visualizing to myself how I would look following chemo. I mentally started to plan my funeral and the worst part of my dilemma was how I would tell my son.

Oh my God! What am I going to do?

♡ Coming to My Spiritual Senses

I want to tell you that there is something unique and enormously powerful about being a woman. There is a certain strength that we have. God has placed in each one of us an extraordinary strength and I believe that no other species on the planet has this strength.

As women, particularly being African American, there is a certain swag, a confident knowing, and an assurance that come what may, we will survive it. Adversity has forced us to be rooted in our faith. We know that life might rock us to our core, but it will not break us. We have a sense of fearlessness not only because we are women, we are fearless, particularly, because we know God.

My grandmother, Alma Woodruff is like many grandmothers. She is a praying, Holy Ghost filled, sanctified woman who will drop a prayer on a dime. She is the epitome of womanhood: strong, virtuous and unwavering. As the cornerstone of our family's spiritual foundation, my grandmother taught me about God and how to trust in the Lord. She taught me that there is power in the name of Jesus. I am sure that her supernatural strength and not to mention her direct dial line to God, spilled over to me on the porch that afternoon in what was a frantic, dark time.

As I stood on the porch in a state of shock, I have to tell you that something so powerful came over me. All of a sudden and in honor the black woman that God made me to be, and yes, I know the correct term is African American. But I use the words "black woman" to emphasize my attitude and conviction as that moment required.

With my hand on my hip; my best neck twist; and a stomp of my foot, I said to God, "Surely, after all that you already brought me through, after all that you have already delivered me from, surely this is not what you intended for my demise. Surely, you did not save me; deliver me--for cancer to kill me. Surely, God in your world this nothing but a pimple so I surrender this to you, and I stand knowing that you will work it out."

The panic that had taken over me had come to an abrupt end. I had come to my spiritual senses.

The panic and fear no longer had a place in my life because I knew with certainty that if God had already delivered me through the worst of times, I knew that God would take care of me in this situation. What I had already come through was in many ways worst than cancer.

Sometimes things come in your life to test your own faith. Not your friends' faith. Not your prayer partner's faith. Not the saints in the church's faith. Not anybody else's faith. God can call you out and God will test your faith.

I knew that in this situation and at this time, if I was going to come out of this adversity: if I was going to survive this at all – I was going to have to stand on my own faith.

Sometimes we live off of other people's faith. In my previous situation, I was surrounded by my sister's faith, my grandmother and her sister's faith, my family's faith, my friend's faith, my prayer partners faith.

My issue was ALWAYS before the altar. The saints were in constant prayer. I was involved in a thirteen-year custody case. My circumstances at that time looked dire. I attended close to sixty custody hearings. I was found in contempt on numerous occasions. And God delivered me out that situation to bring me to cancer? It did not make sense.

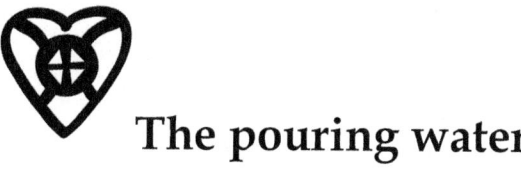# The pouring water

To every thing there is a season,
and a time to every purpose under the heaven.
Ecclesiastes 3:1
King James Version

Decisions, Decisions

After reading the letter on my grandmother's porch I immediately went to God and asked what do you want me to do?

God, what do you want me to do?

Immediately the scripture, Isaiah 58:6 "Is it not the fast that I have commanded of you…to break every yoke?" came into my spirit. I cannot explain it outside of a spiritual understanding but at that point I knew that God was directing my path.

I then called my prayer partner, Deborah and all I said was her name, Deborah. She could tell from the tone of my voice that something was very wrong.

Now let me tell you how God works. He has already given us everything we need –BEFORE WE NEED IT.

My prayer partner is involved in a healing ministry working in the field of drug and alcohol addiction. In 1998, she met a naturopathic healer at one of her conferences. She shared with me the works that this doctor performed but because it did not involve custody issues, I must admit that I half heard her. This was five years before I was diagnosed. God is planning, coordinating, and orchestrating my circumstance even before I knew I had a circumstance. Isn't God awesome?

Now that I had this letter in my hand, I really did not know what to do from a medical point of view. Deborah, a true woman of faith told me that cancer did not mean that it was an automatic death sentence. She suggested that I consult three people: Dr. Frank Miesse, a herbologist in Springfield, Ohio; Dr. Rebecca Glaser, a breast cancer specialist here in Dayton; and Dr. Carlin Browne, a naturopathic doctor in Aruba, the same doctor that she had met five years prior.

I then made the decision to consider all of my options. I wanted to truly make an informed decision. By this point, I was no longer in a panic and neither was I motivated by fear. Spiritually, I began to fast until an answer was made clear.

The first person I consulted was Dr. Rebecca Glaser, a breast cancer specialist here in Dayton, Ohio. She conducted a biopsy and reviewed my mammogram results with me. The tumor in my left breast was in fact very large. The malignant tumor had grown underneath the benign tumor. So, I really could not detect it in my self-examination.

On the mammogram, there was a dark circle in my right underarm pit. But on physical examination, the tumor in the right armpit was no longer there. I had recently had a boil in that arm prior to the mammogram, so that offered a reasonable explanation as to its disappearance. This was an important discovery because it eliminated metastasis as an issue.

Dr. Glaser had a wonderful spirit. She was direct, yet compassionate. I had an immediate connection to her. I sensed that fighting breast cancer was not just her profession, but it was her ministry. She ordered more laboratory test and she arranged for me to meet a breast cancer survivor to serve as my mentor.

The next day, I went to Dr. Frank Miesse in Springfield, Ohio. He is not a medical doctor, but he is highly educated and knowledgeable about herbs and their effect on the body.

By this time, there was much discomfort in my breast. I looked for herbs to strengthen my immune system and improve my overall health. One of the products that I purchased was Paw-Paw by Nature's Sunshine. I took the Paw-Paw along with some other herbs and the pain in my breast lessened.

Dr. Miesse began his examination of me through the science of iridology. Iridology is the study of the body by examining the eyes. Each area of the iris reflects a corresponding part of the body. By looking at the iris, many illnesses are able to be detected.

I spent some time talking with Dr. Miesse about herbal remedies and some of the things he shared with me made a lot of sense. Before I left his office, Dr. Miesse shared one more thing with me. When his wife had breast cancer, she would use castor oil on her breast, and it softened the tumor. Wait, did he say castor oil?

An Unexpected Gift

I returned to Dr. Glaser the following week and I had a lot of decisions to make. I was diagnosed at Stage II and Dr. Glaser felt that I was very treatable. I had tested positive as an estrogen receptor.

Dr. Glaser wanted to proceed with a lumpectomy as well as the removal of a lymph node for testing. There was only one caveat, because of my uncontrollable hypertension, I was deemed a surgical risk and I would have to sign a blanket consent form. I would have to rely on Dr. Glaser's professional judgment during surgery.

I really did not have a problem with that idea, per se, because I liked Dr. Glaser and I trusted her professional judgment. The true red flag in my opinion was the fact that I was deemed a surgical and/or medical risk. That bothered me more than the cancer.

I met with my mentor and she shared her journey with me: the impact of chemotherapy; her faith; and her support system. I am a single mother and at that time, my son was 14 years old. He was not able to drive and he was involved in a situation that required a lot of care and attention. I did not have that type of support system in place for myself, much less for my son. So, I really had to rethink what other options that I could explore.

My biggest concern was not just the cancer, but I was very concerned about my overall health. I wanted to experience wholeness and wellness in all aspects of my life. I had not been very kind to my body. And I was truly bothered by the condition of my health.

The last person on the list that Deborah provided me was Dr. Carlin Browne in Aruba. Prior to contacting Dr. Carlin Browne, I decided to speak to Dr. Frances Brisbane of the State University of New York at Stony Brook. Stony Brook offered a course of study in naturopathic medicine and they had a relationship with Dr. Browne. Students from Stony Brook would go to Aruba for training and Dr. Browne would travel to Stony Brook for lectures and workshops.

I spoke with Dr. Brisbane over the telephone and I expressed my concerns and whether it was feasible to invest in the money to travel to Aruba. Most importantly, I wanted to know exactly who was Carlin Browne? Dr. Brisbane simply said something to the effect that if it were her, Dr. Browne would be the only person that she would see. With this assurance, I then contacted Dr. Carlin Browne.

I shared with Dr. Browne my health status and he asked me if I could come to Aruba. He told me that he thought he could heal me, but I would have to be in Aruba.

Dr. Browne explained to me that he had a machine that would reduce tumors and that he had experienced success in healing people from all over the world. Before we hung up the phone, he offered one last piece of advice: rub your breast with a paste of castor oil and cayenne pepper. Wait another minute, did he say castor oil?

I learned from a friend that castor oil is referred to as the Palma Christi -- the hand of Christ. Pure or cold pressed castor oil traces its roots back some 4,000 years to ancient Egyptian times. It has been used for medicinal purposes to treat a number of aliments. I finally understood Neeka's sense of urgency.

I began to rub my breast in the castor oil and cayenne pepper paste every day. It was the same castor oil that Neeka had insisted that I take home from Jamaica. After the paste was applied, I would wrap my breast in saran wrap and I would pray. I did not know if this castor oil paste was going to work, but I was willing to try.

On my last visit with Dr. Glaser, I spoke to her about my interest in pursuing naturopathic options. She was actually very supportive. Dr. Glaser told me that she believed in healing in any form. For her, healing came through surgery, but she would encourage me to purse whatever course that I was comfortable with. She gave me both freedom and power with these words, *"It is your body and your choice. Don't let anybody take that decision from you."*

I could not believe my ears. It was the first time that I had met a medical doctor who allowed me free rein with my health. And I took it. I will be forever grateful to her for this gift. Because for the rest of my journey, I was in total charge of my health care and I maintained my right to choose what made logical sense to me.

Dr. Glaser had scheduled me for surgery on June 11, 2003. I woke up that morning and canceled the surgery. Within a few days, I was on a plane to Aruba.

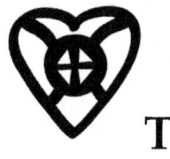 # The soapy brushes

I will lead the blind by a road they do not know,
by paths they have not known I will guide them.
I will turn the darkness before them into light,
the rough places into level ground.
These are the things I will do, and I will not
forsake them.
Isaiah 42:16
NRSV Version

❤ The Way of the Unknown

I must tell you this—I am the least likely person to speak on naturopathic medicine. Prior to this time, the words "holistic medicine" were not in my DNA. I was like Ms. Sophia in the movie, *The Color Purple*, "Y'all can pass the fried chicken" and I like mine with white bread, smashed down with the grease coming out, and sprinkled with hot sauce. So, when I tell you that I am the least likely person to speak about holistic medicine, I **MEAN** that I am the least likely person to say the words. But I came to realize early on that this was a spiritual journey and I was trusting God, all the way to the end.

Up until this point, I have been very quiet about my diagnosis. I had decided not to give it energy with my words. I knew that this situation was a test of my own faith. And because I was walking with God, I felt that God was the only one who I really needed to talk too. I only shared my health with a handful of people--people who I knew were strong in faith. Outside of that small circle, no one else knew.

I was making arrangement to travel to Aruba when I learned that my father was planning a vacation there at the exact same time. I decided to share my health condition with him and my decision to go to Aruba for treatment.

My father offered to wait on me to arrive so that he could go with me to the doctor. To be quite honest, I did not know what type of treatment I was going to receive but, I had this absolute fearlessness about me. The spirit of the Lord was on me because I had such peace.

I was delayed all week on leaving home for Aruba. It was a series of small things that kept getting in the way. Finally, I was scheduled to depart on Saturday afternoon. My flight was to arrive in Atlanta for a 4:00 pm departure to Aruba.

While I was sitting on the plane in Dayton, an announcement came over the loudspeaker stating that there was mechanical failure and we would be delayed. My plane arrived in Atlanta at 3:50 pm. Needless to say, I would not reach Aruba for at least another day.

My father had waited more than a week for me to arrive in Aruba, but his travel plans required him to return home. As my plane was on the way to Aruba, his plane was on the way to Atlanta. And I knew then that my arrival to Aruba alone was intentionally planned by God.

When I checked into my suite at the hotel, I was expecting God to show up at any moment. I opened the patio door and curtains. I thought that the wind was going to blow, and that God was going to come rushing in. But nothing happened, just the sound of the gentle ocean breeze.

After I got settled, I went down to the lobby to inquire about directions and the best method of transportation to Dr. Carlin Browne's Clinica Misericordia. The doorman immediately offered to take me there the next morning. I offered to pay him, and he graciously declined.

On the way to the clinic, I asked him about his generosity, and he said, "When people come to see Dr. Browne, they are usually extremely sick. And I knew that if you were going to see Dr. Browne, I had to help you."

We arrived at Dr. Browne's office in San Nichols. His clinic was on a main fare way. It was a modest two-story building, painted a pale greenish blue. The man explained where I would catch the bus to get back to the hotel. He then called for Dr. Browne. Dr. Browne appeared on the upstairs balcony and he asked me to wait for just one moment. Dr. Browne signaled me to come up the stairs to the balcony. The gentlemen who had been so generous to me waved goodbye and then he departed.

The Miracle in Aruba

When I met Dr. Browne on that balcony, I have never had that type of feeling to come over me, EVER in my life. He had these deep-set eyes and he had this aura over him of complete and absolute peace. If I did not know God, I would have been frightened out of my mind. But I sensed that I was in the presence of God. It was such a quietness and an ease about his spirit. I said to myself, "Okay God, I know that you are here".

We met in a rather large room on the second floor. For a long time, we just sat and talked. We then went downstairs to a very organized office. Because it was Sunday, his secretary was not there. It was just the two of us and we began to bond in a very special, unspoken way.

He explained to me how he treats cancer patients. He told me about some of his success stories and also, some of his challenges. He also began his examination of me through the science of iridology. He then shared with me the exact same thing that Dr. Miesse had shared. He was not worried about cancer as much as he was concerned about the parasites that were consuming my body. Parasites! He explained how parasites invade the body and wreak havoc.

He gave me a diet to follow and he asked that I do everything, exactly as he told me. And I agreed. I left with my instructions. We were to begin treatment the next morning and I could not wait to see how this was going to unfold.

My new diet consisted of fresh fruits and vegetables, absolutely no meat or dairy. The next morning, I prepared the meals as Dr. Browne had directed: the juice of six limes mixed with olive oil; *Very Nasty*.

Next, I had one apple slowly cooked, mixed with oatmeal and topped off with black strap molasses. *Unconsciously Nasty*. I cannot even describe how nasty this tasted. There are simply no words. It was almost impossible to swallow, thick and bitter. But I had made the commitment to wholeness so there was no turning back now.

I arrived early at Dr. Browne's. After eating the breakfast that he had directed, I was prepared for anything. I was greeted, softly, by Dr. Browne. His continence was always soft and gentle. His nurse, Patricia Hall was in the office and with her by his side, Dr. Browne began to conduct a thorough examination.

Dr. Browne clinic was in fact a mini compound. There were a series of three small outbuildings that surrounded the main building. The clinic was designed with the Stony Brook

University interns in mind. It was also designed to accommodate a limited number of critical patients.

After my examination, I went to one of the adjacent buildings to begin my treatment. The first stop was in the reflexology room. I had never participated in reflexology prior to this time. I understood some aspects to it, but I did not know how much it HURT! The gentleman who served as the reflexologist only spoke Spanish. And I later grew to appreciate how skilled he was. But this first encounter was unbearable. I thought that it hurt worst than childbirth.

I learned that in reflexology, very much like iridology, each of the body's organs and systems have a corresponding location on both the feet and the hands. Because of the condition of my breast, each time the reflexologist touched the corresponding area on my foot, I would literally holler.

After reflexology, I moved across the hall to another room. This room contained the light machine that Dr. Browne had spoken of. I never knew the name of this machine, but I have spent years trying to track it down.

The machine was oblong in shape and it emitted infra red lights. It was placed directly above the tumor and the light would beam down. It did not externally burn the skin, although you could feel the heat. I would stay under this light machine for about two hours.

After the light machine and reflexology, I would return to the main building for additional treatment.

Some days I would have acupuncture. One day Dr. Browne wrapped my breast with a clay mixture that had a drawing effect. One another day, Dr. Browne injected the tumor with some mixture that had a bubbling, tingly sensation. Some days I would stay all day long. Sometimes I would come to the clinic in the early morning. Sometimes I would come in the evening, which was really good because it allowed me to see Aruba. Some days I was required to swim in the ocean so that the salt water could help with the healing. Dr. Browne was an advocate of rest. He took afternoon naps, daily. And some days, I also rested.

Over the course of treatment, I found out quite a bit about Dr. Browne. He was at least in his late 80's to early 90's, if not older. I based this calculation on the stories he told.

Carlin Browne was born on an indigenous island off the coast of Aruba. His mother was the village midwife. The doctor visited the island only twice a year. According to Dr. Browne, his mother kept an amazing record of everyone she treated. Not only did she keep records about those she treated but she was careful to record every remedy she used as well as every response to the remedy.

Initially, Dr. Browne had no interest in medicine. He pursued a number of careers including law. But it was his own near-death experience that led him to seek out his mother's old remedies. Dr. Browne then made naturopathic medicine his life's work with training in the Netherlands, Germany and Asia. He was both a Medical Doctor and a Doctor of Naturopathic Medicine.

I learned so much about the body from Dr. Browne. And I have adopted many of his beliefs. The first and foremost is that the body was designed by God to heal itself. I truly believe this. And the other belief is that in creating the Earth, God made an abundance of herbs for the body's natural healing process. And again, I believe this to be true. But beyond my beliefs, the most compelling aspect of my treatment was the complete metamorphosis of my own body.

When I arrived in Aruba, the tumor in my left breast was the size of an orange and it had no movement. My breast tissue was hard. There was no bounce or sponge in it. And my skin was stiff like leather. Within a week, the tumor began to shrink. My tissue was becoming spongy again and I felt absolutely wonderful.

Dr. Browne was encouraged by my response. He was hopeful that he could completely eradicate the tumor but because of its size, he felt that I needed some additional time.

As I mentioned before, I was involved in a lengthy and intense custody situation and I had a hearing schedule on July 2, 2003. I did not have the liberty with the court to post-pone the hearing. I *had* to return to the United States. If I had revealed to the court that I was dealing with breast cancer, I believe that it would have been used against me. I was faced with choosing my own life or the life and well-being of my son. I am a mother — so I chose my son's life over my own.

I returned from Aruba with a new breast and a new outlook on cancer. The orange that had been in my breast was now down to the size of a walnut. I continued the herbal remedies that Dr. Browne had prescribed. I continued to seek other naturopathic options as well. At this point in my life, I was **SOLD.** There was no way that I would ever consider anything else.

❤ The Holistic Way

Some twenty years before I made this commitment to wholeness and wellness, I was living in the Washington, DC area and I met Alan Price. He is a dear friend of my sister Monica and at that time, they both race-walked. Alan holds the one hundred miles U.S. record in race-walking, and he was a big proponent for natural living.

He, along with my sister, would encourage me to race-walk with them. Alan would also encourage me to change my high carbohydrate diet. I ignored him on the diet thing, and I did not, under any circumstances, ever consider walking to the corner much less engage in competitive walking. But I was supportive, and I would often go to their practices and watch.

I heard Alan when he spoke about having a holistic lifestyle but that was for him, it was not for me. This is another example of how God is planning, orchestrating, and coordinating my life path.

Upon my return from Aruba, I contacted Alan and I shared with him my new conversion as well as my conviction to natural living. He also shared with me some of the herbs and products that were making an impact on cancer treatment.

Throughout my journey, I have consulted and relied on Alan's knowledge. I have not made any decisions about my natural healthcare without speaking to him. He has never guided me in the wrong direction.

I was able to find some naturopathic support in the Dayton area. From time to time, I would go back to see Dr. Miesse and restock on herbs. I also found another practitioner who gave me guidance. I tried a number of options such as being wrapped in foil and zapped. It is one of those things that are truly sci-fi and if I did not experience it directly, there is no way I would believe it.

In the naturopathic community, it is a big belief that diseased bodies are infected with parasites. It is believed that the parasites influence the course of the disease. So, in theory if you kill the parasites, you can circumvent the illness.

I understood the logic of what they were saying, and I did not doubt that parasites can invade and infect the body, but I was skeptic. Because I was new to this journey in wellness, I was open to try many things that I would not have ordinarily considered. However, I was not so desperate that I would try anything. The course of treatment had to be compelling.

This new practitioner suggested that I undergo a zapping process to get rid of the parasites. I was wrapped in an aluminum foil sheet.

Everything was covered except the opening of my nose and my mouth. I held two electric probes and I waited for something to happen. After about 20 minutes, nothing happened.

I was miserable because my entire body was wrapped. I thought this particular practitioner was crazy and that this was really a gimmick. It was my first visit with this practitioner, and I reasoned that it was definitely going to be my last: just as soon as they unwrapped me, I was OUT-OF-THERE. Another 20 minutes passed and still nothing. The practitioner came in the room and quietly began to pray.

All of a sudden, my body began to itch and tinkle. It was the parasites. They were coming out of my ears, out of my legs, out of my arms, out of my abdomen. And as they were coming out of me, you could hear the crinkling of the foil sheet.

Just like the bugs that you zap in your backyard, the parasites that had invaded my body were being zapped. In the zapping process, the electric probes emit a high-pitched radio frequency that only the parasites can hear, very much like the invisible fence that people use for their pets. The connection to the invisible fence actually made sense to me as well as what I had just witness in my own body.

From October 2003 to 2006, I began to frequent this practitioner for my natural health care needs. Over the years, we have developed a good friendship.

In addition to my local practitioner, I kept in telephone contact with Dr. Browne. I tried in every way that I could to get back to Aruba for treatment. I learned in January 2005 that Dr. Browne had passed on Christmas Eve. I was heartbroken.

The side to side pounding of the heavy wet rags

The rain fell, the floods came, and the winds blew and beat on the house, but it did not fall, because it had been founded on rock.
Matthew 7:25
NRSV Version

The Big, the Bad and the Ugly

In spite of my faith and even though I had adopted a holistic lifestyle, the tumor continued to grow. I cannot adequately describe the pain that I endured for more than three years--the fire, the burning, and the intense sting. The tumor was so aggressive that it began to eat from the inside to the outside of my body. I had both an internal tumor and an external tumor. The gravity of this situation is difficult to explain. My breast was split opened and you could physically see the brown tar-like tumor as well as the yellowish pus like flesh. The tumor looked like brown cauliflower clusters coming right out of my breast.

By February 2006, I was in so much pain. I knew that I had to do something. I could not continue to exist with my breast open. Even though I was opposed to chemotherapy, the intense pain that I was experiencing made me reconsider my options.

I was without health insurance, having been dropped by my insurance carrier. I had exhausted all of my savings on my health care. I was living on the internet at this time trying to find programs that could help me.

I stumbled upon the Cancer Prevention Institute website and to my surprise; it was located in my hometown. I contacted their office and spoke with an angel, Kathy Haught. She listened to my story and she asked a lot of questions. She told me about a program that would cover all of the cost of my breast cancer treatment. This program, the Breast and Cervical Cancer Project (BCCP), was available to low income women. I immediately relinquished my income so that I could be eligible to enroll in this program.

From a medical perspective, the BCCP is a Godsend. It is a federal program which is administered by various states. It allows poor and low-income women to receive full cancer treatment. Surgery, including reconstruction, chemotherapy, radiation, mammograms, MRI's, PET scans and medication are all covered under this program. Kathy, who is a nurse and the BCCP Program Manager, was very knowledgeable about cancer prevention and treatment. She provided me with a list of physicians who worked with patients in the program. The physician that I was scheduled to see had actually taken over Dr. Glaser's practice, so my previous medical records were readily available.

I met with this particular surgeon in mid-February. My breast was significantly opened by this time. This surgeon, like Dr. Glaser, specialized solely in the treatment of breast cancer. She immediately referred me to a local medical oncologist. The surgeon explained that in my current condition I was not able to have a mastectomy, the tumor was too large. It was suggested that I follow a course in chemotherapy and then have the mastectomy.

I was in surrender at this time. I was talking to God constantly. In my heart, I did not desire chemotherapy, but I was willing to go wherever God took me. Plus, the pain was so compelling.

I met with the medical oncologist on Wednesday, February 22, 2006. He was interested in my story and respected my decision to first seek naturopathic options. He was not critical.

He explained in detail what I was going to go through. Very much the same as my mentor had shared with me in 2003. But this time instead of an all-out rejection of chemotherapy, I was at least willing to give it a try. My heart, my mind, my soul was truly saddened, but I was living in a surrendered body and I had a surrendered life; "Not my will Father but your will be done."

We had an intense discussion about traditional verses naturopathic options in cancer treatment. This particular doctor did not totally reject naturopathic options, but he was a proponent of traditional treatment options. He was easy to talk to and if I were going to go through this process, I believed that I would be in good hands.

He asked two things of me. One, refrain from the use of herbs during the course of the chemotherapy and two, could he photograph my open breast and present my case to his colleagues. I said yes to both requests.

I was scheduled for all kinds of test including an MRI and a PET scan. While I was in his office, my blood work was drawn. I was going to begin my first chemotherapy treatment on Wednesday, March 8, 2006.

The doctor suggested that I have a port place in my chest to ease the administration of the chemo. I did not want the port, but he explained that the chemo combination that I was going to have would burn a hole if it came in contact with my skin. Bells and alarms were ringing in my head but unless God changed my plans, this was going to be my path.

I went to Kettering Medical Center on Wednesday, March 1, 2006 for my pre-op test, chest x-ray and EKG. I was to return on Monday, March 6, 2006 for surgery to have the port inserted in my chest.

I was sitting at my desk on Friday, March 3, 2006 and my phone rang. I could tell from the number that the call was from the hospital. The lady on the other end informed me that they were going to have to cancel my surgery scheduled for Monday. The EKG showed that there was a blockage in my heart, and I was not medically able to have chemotherapy at this time.

I was about to jump right out of my chair, not from fear but from joy. There is a song that comes on the radio, *Jesus Can Work It Out*, and I was stomping my feet underneath my desk and my soul was singing, *"work it out"*.

The lady informed me that I would have to have clearance from a cardiologist before they could continue. I hung up the phone and I SHOUTED. It was confirmation that God had another plan for me, and I was going to watch him work it out.

♥ Working It Out

The following Wednesday, March 8, 2006 when my chemotherapy appointment came around, I debated on whether or not I should go. I was not going to be able to start the treatment, but I liked and respected the doctor enough that I thought I would keep the appointment.

When the doctor arrived in the examination room, he was upbeat and excited about my first chemotherapy treatment. He had not been informed about the medical hold. He said, "Well since you are here, let's take a look at your test results".

He told me that I was at Stage III. My brain was clear, my lungs were clear, my liver was clear. Then he said, "The most amazing thing has happened. Your tumor marker came back normal."

I did not know what that meant. I was thinking that maybe the size of my tumor was normal for where I was in staging. So, I asked if he measured the tumor.

He replied, "No".

He went on to explain that the tumor maker measures your blood and the amount of cancer that is in the blood. Mine came back normal; the cancer was not showing up in my blood!

The doctor went on to say, "You know, for as long as you have been dealing with this thing, your tumor marker should be off the chart. I am truly amazed at your results."

I left his office and I went to see my grandmother. As I mentioned previously, she is saved, and Holy Ghost filled. When I explained to her what the doctor said, we shouted and Holy Ghost danced in her living room until we were exhausted. In my grandmother's tears she said something so profound. She said, "You know Rhonda, God is so good that sometimes you can just taste Him." Now that is some God!

I could not ignore what was happening before my very eyes. This was further confirmation that I was on a spiritual journey even though it appeared in the form of a medical issue.

I followed up with the cardiologist and I went through a series of test. On March 31, 2006, I was cleared by my cardiologist. No blockage.

I took advantage of this medical information: tumor marker normal and no blockage. I was more determined than ever to chart my own course. I was constantly on the internet looking for solutions that I could live with. I found out about this procedure called Radiofrequency Ablation (RFA) and I wanted to give this a try.

I do not want to seem as if I was just wishing and fishing for *any* solution. I *knew* that I had experience positive results in Aruba. In spite of the size of the tumor, I *knew* that the herbs were effective in keeping me alive. I always looked for a natural option as close as possible to my Aruba experience.

I contacted a radiologist in Cincinnati and made an appointment to see him. He was energetic and somewhat enthused. He was interested in my case from a medical perspective because I was in such good shape. I presented him with the opportunity for additional medical research. At this doctor's urging, I made an appointment with another breast cancer specialist.

A Heavy Blow

During the three years of dealing with cancer, I had been to every doctor's visit and to every procedure alone. My family was concerned and my sister Monica, my niece and my son accompanied me on this visit. My sister asked if she could come in the examination room with me. I had hand-carried all of my medical records so that there would be no delay in deciding if Radiofrequency Ablation could be used in my situation.

As soon as the doctor entered into the room, our spirits collided. It was an all-out battle. She took a courtesy look at my breast and then she spoke, "You have no chance or no possibility of surviving this."

She continued, "You have willfully put yourself in this position by your misdirected use of alternative medicine. Your breast is wide open. You started at Stage II. You have allowed this to reach Stage IV. There is not anything that anybody can do to help you at this point. The most that can happen is that we can make you comfortable."

Just like that: blunt and to the point.

My sister gasped.

I was angered by her demeanor and by her tone. The fact that she told me that I was going to die did not hurt nearly as bad as her reprimand and her judgment in my use of naturopathic medicine.

I think what I found so frustrating was this belief that my pursuit of naturopathic medicine was an act of negligence on my part. I have always realized that my non-traditional approach to treatment would not be embraced or accepted by everyone. But her tone was not merely a rejection of my choice, it was a direct assault.

As I have explained to everyone who asked about my decision to reject traditional cancer treatment, I did not act purely from an emotional perspective. I read. I researched. I asked questions. I prayed. And having made sure that I was able to be informed as much as possible, I then followed what made logical and spiritual sense to me.

I felt compelled to defend my choice. In retrospect, I should have simply smiled.

This doctor continued, as if the first blow were not enough. "I don't care what anybody else tells you. I don't care if your tumor marker was normal or not. You have to realize that you are going to die. You need to grow up and accept your fate."

I kindly followed her advise and responded as a grown up should. I told her that *if* I was going to die, then I was going to do it my way. And she could rest assured that she would not facilitate that process. If I was dying, I knew with certainty that this doctor would not have a thing to do with my death.

With my renewed energy, I gathered my clothing and I thanked her for her time. I was actually happy to depart from her presence, death sentence and all.

When we got into the lobby, my sister Monica asked me, "What are we going to do now?" Still seething in anger, I told her that "we" are not going to do anything. "I" was going to continue to trust God.

My sister looked at me as if to say, 'didn't you hear her?'

I responded, "Yes, I heard her but that is *her* truth, it is not *my* truth. I am standing on God's word that with his stripes I am already healed. That *is* my only truth".

The elevator door opened, and it was as if I was stepping into a new life. I was beyond angry at the doctor's lack of compassion as well as her lack of decorum. It was a turning point for me in a way. I was more determined than EVER to live. I was going back to show her how very wrong she was. This became my unspoken drive, "God will prove her wrong."

♥ Big Girls Don't Cry

The thing about facing death is that it can play on your mind. No matter how cool or composed I may have been on the outside, my head was going through changes.

For the next few months, every night that I went to bed, I wondered, "Is this the night that I am going to die?" The thought of dying was constantly on my mind. Each morning as I awaken, I would look at the sunlight and wondered if I was in heaven. Even after my eyes were fully opened, I would pinch myself to see if I was still alive. This went on for awhile and the anger continued to brew.

One day I decided that I had had enough. I came to the realization that we all face a certain death, but *I was not dead.* At that moment, I made the conscious decision to live. I was going to live until I died. I *mean* I was going to live every moment to the fullest. I was going to squeeze every drop that life had to offer. And if and when I died, life was not going to owe me *ANYTHING.*

I began to awake each morning with a new drive and determination. I was consciously choosing life. Each morning I would say, "I choose life. This is a great day to be alive." I came to both the realization and to the acceptance that God had purposed my life. There was to be no whining or no complaining. With God's help, I was going to press my way through this experience.

My family and my friends were extremely supportive, but they were also very frightened. They quietly disagreed with my belief system. They could not understand why I was so opposed to chemotherapy because they could not see any outer change in my medical condition. Many wondered how I could just ignore what the doctor had said and why I was not doing something.

What they could not see in the outer being, I completely understood inwardly. I asked them not to agree with my decision. I did not want them to even try to understand my decision. All I wanted was for them to respect my choice. Whatever the outcome, I owned it.

I knew that I was on a spiritual journey. I knew that I was somehow being used by God. I tried to explain this, but it seemed like it was difficult for people to conceive. As people, we talk about God all of the time. We quote scriptures from the bible with ease. At that time, I did not know the word of God all that well, but I knew, that God was directing my life. Even if I could not articulate it, I understood it.

♥ Searching for the Light

From a medical perspective, I continued to seek naturopathic treatment. I was still taking a lot of herbs. I was still looking for "the light" that I had found in Aruba.

One day my friend Deborah called and asked about the light. She wanted me to describe it to her. Deborah told me that she had visited a lady's home and she had "the light" right here in Dayton.

In August 2006, I met Rose and I began going to her house for treatment. The light was called the Beam Ray. It was a version of the machine made by Royal Rife. This light emitted ultraviolet rays through a radio frequency, just like the zapper. The frequency was set at a pitch that would destroy cancer cells.

Royal Rife was a scientist who invented a high-powered microscope that could see and destroy microorganisms. This microscope could destroy the microorganisms by emitting a light through high frequency pitches. When the light frequency reached a certain pitch, the microorganism was destroyed. Royal Rife conducted human trials during the 1930's and was successful with the destruction of cancer cells and other pathogens.

I did this treatment twice a day for about one and a half hours each time. Now how did I know that it was working? Each time the light would go through its flash cycle, my left breast would throb and pound. When the light cycle was stable, the breast would immediately stop pounding.

Rose was an absolute angel. Professionally, she worked as a nurse for more than thirty years and she was committed to total wellness. Rose did not charge one dime for the use of the Beam Ray. After a few months, she allowed me to take one her Beam Ray's home.

I used this Beam Ray for several months and I absolutely loved it. One day I plan on purchasing this machine. Although the tumor did not get smaller, I am convinced that the destruction of other microorganisms in my body help to sustain me.

My left breast was open and each time my cycle started; I would have an eruption in the tumor. One night while I was using the Beam Ray, I had an eruption. As the flash cycle began, blood gushed everywhere. I decided to end my use of the Beam Ray until I could get a hold on the bleeding.

My niece Rhea was not frightened by the bleeding. She was the only one in my household who was able to help me. Sometimes the bleeding would be so bad that I would stand over the sink and just let the blood pour out. I learned that cayenne pepper immediately stops bleeding

59

anywhere in the body. Someone would have to run to the kitchen and get the pepper and hot water. I would drink it like a tea. The bleeding would stop immediately. This profuse bleeding started in January 2007 and continued through March 2008.

My family would plead with me to go to the hospital each time I had an eruption. I refused to go because I knew that no one would understand my ways.

By January 2008, I was battle weary. No matter how strong your faith is, there does come a point when you just feel as though you cannot take anymore. The tumor was larger than it ever had been. I had a secondary tumor in my left lymph node that was the size of an ostrich egg. The smell of my open flesh was unbearable. I would cleanse my wound with a peroxide bath. I would then take surgical gauze and apply Vaseline on the gauze. I placed this Vaseline gauze directly over my wound.

The wound would drain onto the gauze. Within a few hours, the gauze was complete soaked. I had to change my dressing three to four times a day.

I went to see a doctor friend of mine who was a wound specialist. When she saw my breast she said, "You know that you should not be alive. Not only the cancer, but the bacteria in your open wound should have killed you a long time ago."

She told me to get some raw sugar in the packet and pour it directly on the wound. Almost immediately, the dead and rotten flesh began to slough off. And the smell began to die down.

At this particular time, I was in an inconceivable and an unconscionable amount of pain. The amount of physical suffering that I endured is difficult to explain and even more difficult to believe.

During this entire process, I refused to take narcotics, of any form. I did take 800 mg of Ibuprofen as often as I could to take the edge off of the pain. I am truly a demonstrated case of mind over matter. I could not in my mind, live in my affliction. I could not imagine just lying in pain and waiting to die. And I knew that if I surrendered to the pain, that I would not be able to fight. I knew that I had to stay alert, my life and my faith were depending upon my will to live.

The intense heat showed up and everything dried

*I consider that the sufferings of this present time
are not worthy comparing
with the glory about to be revealed to us.*
Romans 8:18
NRSV Version

63

The Valley of Job

In the bible God asks Satan not once but twice, *"Hast thou considered my servant Job?"* As a Christian, I knew the story of Job. I had endured a lot of heartache during my life. I lost my mother when I was in my early twenties. I had come through a horrific divorce. I had supported my child through many challenges that were beyond his control. I had never compared myself to Job. As things came at me, I just developed a tougher skin and I learned how to live off just sheer will.

I also learned to appreciate my past hurts because it really gave me a foundation for perseverance. But no matter how solid a foundation that I was standing on, nothing prepared me for what I was about to encounter.

It is one thing to face a catastrophic health situation. It is a whole other thing to face a catastrophic financial situation. But to have them show up at the same time...

Because of my lack of health insurance, I elected to go into an income limiting program that would provide me with the necessary medical coverage. I had acquired some savings but because I had been "self-pay" during all my years of medical care, those resources dried quickly.

I thought that I could make it for a few months with no income at least until the treatment was over. Once my treatment was over, I knew that I could return to full time employment. My son was entering his senior year in high school and within a few months we were looking for a place to live. It was as if a wrecking ball was swinging in every direction. Before I could get my footing, there was one collapse after another.

I found myself with no money, no income and basically no place to live. I was never forced to live on the street, but I was not in control of my living situation. I was living at the mercy and kindness of others.

I was forced to live within the public welfare system. In some ways, it is an area of much shame. Here I was college educated and my health condition rendered me unemployable. It was truly a desert experience.

Just like watching a house burn, everything I had worked for was gone. By February 2008, I no longer had a car. I needed to take care of some business and I had no money and no transportation. My sister Monica had become my full-time caregiver at this point. She told me that she was on her way to pick me up. And then, something hit me.

Take Up Thy Bed and Walk

My spirit told me not to wait on her. I was directed to "just get up and walk". I called my sister back and told her not to pick me up; I was going to walk to my appointment. She insisted that I wait on her, but I told her that I was going to be fine.

It was another turning point in my healing. I started walking on this bitter cold February morning. My appointment was about three miles away. I was physically out of shape so walking to the corner was a challenge. But I walked on. Step by step, I walked.

It took me a little more than an hour to reach my destination, but I had made it. I did not realize it at the time that this act of obedience was about to change everything in me.

For the rest of the year, I walked just about everywhere that I needed to go. In most instances, I refused to ride the bus and I refused to accept rides. I would walk five to seven miles every day. I was on a journey and the walking was taking me there. Where the "there" was, I did not know but I was on the move.

Walking became my sanctuary. It was the one place that I could lose myself in the Lord. My family and my friends would pass me on the street, and they would offer me a ride. I would smile and wave them on. Most of the times they felt hurt and I am sure that in a way, they felt sorry for me. But they did not know that I was not in any way defeated. I was smiling on the inside. With every step that I was taking, I was thanking the Lord. I was in full praise with every step and with every breath.

I was pushing past all obstacles and limitations. I was pushing past every hurt and every lost. I was alive and I was thriving. I was walking in my victory.

 # A little light emerges

The people walking in darkness
have seen a great light; on those living
in the land of deep darkness
a light has dawned.
Isaiah 9:2
New International Version

♥ Things Hoped For

Two things happened in my life that I found so encouraging.   I met Dr. Ruth Lavigne, a radiologist oncologist and I found a church to worship and grow in.

I found Dr. Lavigne through an internet search.   A friend of mine had shared with me a website that someone had sent to her. The website was www.howibeatcancer.com. There was a picture of a man with a tumor coming out of the side of his face that was surreal. If I did not have the same tumor coming out of the side of my breast, I would have immediately dismissed the picture as trick photography.   This man photographed his progression throughout his treatment. He began treatment in February 2007 and by September 2007, the tumor was completely gone. I always had faith, now I had hope.

The treatment that this man followed was called tomotherapy.   Tomotherapy is a form of radiation that targets a specific tumor. The surrounding tissue and organs are not impacted by the radiation.

I looked online to see what places in Ohio offered this type of cancer treatment. One of the hospitals was Cleveland Clinic which is about three hours from my home. Precision Radiology in West

Chester was the other. West Chester is only 45 minutes away from me. And I figured that if this was not going to work, I only lost 45 minutes.

I made an appointment to see Dr. Ruth Lavigne. I was excited about the possibility of having this huge tumor protruding out of my breast eliminated. I could not wait to get there.

As soon as I met Dr. Lavigne, I had this sense that I was going to be okay. She had a calm spirit. We were close in age and both of us were mothers. We chatted for awhile. She genuinely wanted to know all about my journey and how I arrived at this point. She listened tentatively as I provided her with my physical, emotional, and psychological perspective.

I shared with her my belief in naturopathic medicine. I told her of my reluctance to take chemotherapy. I shared with her my interest in tomotherapy. This was all done before my physical examination began.

When Dr. Lavigne saw my breast, the panic look on her face said it all. She fell short of releasing a gasp, but her professionalism allowed her composure to be maintained. By this point, my breast was about fifty percent split open with pus like drainage that was pretty bad. The tumor consumed about ninety percent of my breast. Because of the tumor's weight and size, I could not lift my hand over my head. And I know that

Dr. Lavigne probably wanted to say that there was no hope and no possibility, but she did not.

To break the silence and also, to set the tone of why I was there, I opened my mouth and simply said, "I want you to know that I am not afraid to die. Death does not scare me, but right now I want to live. So, what I want to know from you is whether or not you can help me to live?"

She replied, "We are certainly going to try."

The first thing that Dr. Lavigne did was to reassure me that she was going to do everything within her power to help me. Next, she told me that tomotherapy was not an option for me at this time. The tumor was simply too large. She then ordered a series of test to see where I was medically and scheduled me to return to her office within the week.

Before leaving her office that day, she walked with me to the lobby where my sister Monica was waiting. She told my sister that they were going to take good care of me. She hugged me and gave me that same reassurance.

You Don't Make Medical Sense

I was scheduled for a CAT scan, MRI, PET scan, and mammogram at Kettering Memorial Hospital in Dayton. Because my breast was opened, I could not get the mammogram on the left breast. I returned to Dr. Lavigne's office the following week.

My results came back with advance cancer in the left breast. Also, they saw a "hot spot" on my right rear rib which would have confirmed that the cancer had spread. I heard her about the rib, but I was focused on the breast particularly because it caused me so much discomfort. I was not willing to give energy to the possibility of the cancer being in the rib because if it showed up in the rib, it was theoretically everywhere else in my body. And I simply could not take that on.

Dr. Lavigne sent me upstairs to have a consultation with a medical oncologist to see what he would recommend. I met with this doctor for about an hour. He did a physical exam as well and then we talked. He said, "You don't make medical sense."

He continued, "If you were my patient five years ago and had refused chemotherapy, I would have told you that you would not be alive in five years, yet here you are today, still living." He sent me back downstairs to Dr. Lavigne without clear directions as to what to do. He was truly baffled.

When I returned to Dr. Lavigne's office, she spoke with me in her consultation room. It was very relaxed and very peaceful in that room. She began to tell me that she agreed with the prior physician in that I did not "make medical sense". She was not sure what course of action would be best. This was not based upon her medical knowledge, but she was sensitive to my belief system and my complete opposition to traditional chemotherapy.

She explained that in treating me, she did not want to create this power struggle, a tug-of-war, so to speak that if she recommended a course of treatment and I rejected it, we would not accomplish anything.

I immediately said to her, "Dr. Lavigne, surely you don't think that this is a medial issue."

I continued, "Yes, I know of the diagnosis. Yes, I see the tumor hanging out of my breast. This cannot be physiological because if it were, I would not be alive. This is spiritual and it has nothing to do with me and it has nothing to do with you. God has preserved me; God has purposed my life and I stand on God's word that I am healed. The physical manifestation of my healing may not have taken place but when God takes me to the place and when he brings the people into my life that are ordained to

75

be a part of my healing, then the tumor and the cancer in my body will be no more".

The tears began to well in Dr. Lavigne's eyes.

I understood that my situation was outside of the natural realm because I had defied all medical logic. I had lived with "active cancer" for five years at this point. Even though I was in the worst physical pain that I had ever experienced in my life, I still had so much fight in me, and I had this strong will to live. I understood that this was just a moment of time in my life. I had endured so much up until this point that I was not going to allow this situation to swallow me. I knew that this too, shall pass.

I think that my attitude and my disposition had an effect on Dr. Lavigne as well. I was not just talking fearlessness; I was truly living it.

The conversation then became more personal. Dr. Lavigne shared with me her own belief in naturopathic medicine when needed. I so appreciated her honesty because up until this point, almost every traditional doctor that I saw, rejected the notion of naturopathic medicine.

Dr. Lavigne wanted to find a balance between what I believed and what I would tolerate. She suggested that I go see a colleague, also in the Cincinnati area. She knew him professionally and after twenty-five years as a medical oncologist, he had just opened a naturopathic practice. This was truly music to my ears. She gave me a prescription for Tamoxifen because she said that it would address what she suspected was a hormonal issue.

Dr. Lavigne ordered two additional tests. A core biopsy of my breast as well as a biopsy of my right rear rib. I was to return to her office in a couple of weeks.

I made an appointment to see this doctor. He made a combination of Chinese herbs for me to take. I asked about the Tamoxifen and he felt that the Tamoxifen would be okay as well. He made only one recommendation; do not take the herbs with the Tamoxifen. Take one or the other but not both. That way, I would know if and what, I was responsive too. Of course, I took the Chinese herbs.

Within in twenty-four hours, the tumor shrunk significantly. I took the herbs for about one month until I ran out. I did not have money to continue with the herbs, so I then took the Tamoxifen. By the time I started the Tamoxifen, the tumor was half its size and it continued to shrink. Halleluiah!

The Power in Pause

I also had the core biopsy on my breast. I went by myself as I had done on several other occasions. My sister Monica had asked me if I wanted her to go with me, but I declined. I did not think much of it. This was in early March 2008 and it was still bitter cold outside.

I arrived at the outpatient clinic and they called me back to the procedure room. I put on the hospital gown, laid back and waited for the procedure to begin. The nurse came in and prepped me. She injected my breast with anesthesia to numb it and then the doctor came in. Because my breast was open, it presented a challenge. The biopsy had to be taken from underneath the tumor.

Due to the sheer size of the tumor, they were not able to numb me at all. But no one knew that fact until the doctor cut me open. I thought I was going to die right there on that table. I screamed to the top of my lungs and the nurse tried to inject me again, but it was still non-effective.

Because I was cut open, the doctor proceeded on. She inserted that core gun into the opening and began to clip my tissue. Psychologically, I can still feel the pain as she clicked, clicked, clicked away. I have never been a fan of a core biopsy because

I do not like the sound of the biopsy gun. But in this case, I could feel every push and tug.

Both the nurse and doctor were apologetic but in retrospect, I should have been sedated because the pain was unreal. When I went to the lobby to retrieve my coat, I was bent completely to my left side. I could not straighten upright.

The women in the lobby had a panic look on their face. I know that they heard my screams and now they saw my visible pain. I am sure they thought, *'I am not going back there'*. They helped me put on my coat. I wobbled out of there to get the car. I did not know how I was going to drive. I did not know how I was going to make it home. I hurt that bad.

I managed to give my sister a call and she met me as I was pulling up. She helped me out of the car and got me settled in bed. I could not even cry. The tears just rolled down my cheeks.

The most interesting thing happened in this process, I became silent. I mean I was not able to talk. It hurt just to open my mouth. For three weeks I stayed in the bed unable to talk or move. I cancelled the rib biopsy because I could not deal with anymore pain. I was already forced to sleep on my back and there was no way I was willing to have my back compromised. Also, from a spiritual perspective, I knew that as a woman, I was made from the rib of man and I just did not think that the rib was something I should mess with.

I began to talk to God to try to get an understanding of what was going on in my life. I had always talked to God, but this was different. I was going to turn fifty in a few weeks and this silence had forced me to look inward.

I had no money. I had no income. I had no place of my own to live. I was fighting a life-threatening illness and I needed to find my way back to myself. This was not a pity party; I do not believe in them. This was a time for true reflection and introspective.

I did not need to know the why; I needed to know the what. What is it that God wanted from me? What did God want from my life? I was physically silent but spiritually, I was very much alive.

⟡ It's a Spiritual Thing

Long before my diagnosis there was a group of women who prayed for me and my son. My sister Monica was in a prayer ministry on her job. This prayer group would meet during lunch and my sister presented my situation to the group and asked for their prayers.

For thirteen years, this group of women kept my son and me on their prayer list. In 2008, my sister ran into one of the members, Barbara Pinson, in the store. Barbara asked my sister about the "little boy" named Carson. My sister told her that he was now nineteen years old and, on his way, back to college. My sister told her how much Carson was thriving and how his life had been turned around. She then told Barbara about my health situation and she again asked Barbara for her prayers. This was on a Saturday afternoon.

The following Tuesday, Barbara called my sister and said that she had spoken to the other ladies in the group and they wanted to have a special prayer with me at her house on Saturday. I had never met these women, yet they had prayed for my son and me, without ceasing.

I was in the height of my illness at this time. I was in an unconscionable amount of pain. The tumor had grown so large that I could not reach my arm over my head to comb my hair. I was in so much pain that if you just brushed by my left side, I would cringe. One night the pain was so severe that my sister literally rocked me to sleep. Sometimes the pain was so bad that tears would just freely flow down my cheeks.

Throughout my illness I never complained. I just endured. I decided to always find the good in the situation. The amazing thing was that I rarely felt ill. My primary complaint was the excruciating pain. I used to speak to my dear friend Carman often. She is an amazing person in her own right because during my illness she had a heart transplant. Yet she took the time to check on me as often as possible. I would tell her, "Carman, if I can get past the pain, I will be alright."

On this particular week, I was battling flu-like symptoms. I did not have the energy to go anywhere, but I felt compelled to go to the prayer meeting. The least I could do was to tell them thank you.

I arrived at the prayer meeting and there I met these ladies for the first time. Among them were Barbara Pinson, Mother Betty Barnett, Charlette Franklin, and others. I told them about my journey with Carson and how well he was doing. I told them about my faith in dealing with the cancer. I thanked them for all of their years of prayer. Then they prayed with me.

After the prayer meeting, there was fellowship and talking. Mother Betty was speaking about her church and how much she loved it there. Another lady chimed in and agreed. I asked them what church they attended, and the lady answered, "Greater Love Christian Church."

I was not familiar with this church by its name, so I asked where was it located? She told me that it was on the corner of Lakeview and Clifton, the old St. Luke and I smiled.

About ten days before this prayer meeting, one of my former students was shot and killed. He was the first homicide victim in 2008. My sister Monica and I agreed to go and pay our respect, but we did not plan to stay for the funeral. We were in separate cars and we did not see one another there.

As I was about to leave, Cheryl Wood, a classmate from high school walked in the door. I was surprised to see her as I did not know that she knew this young man and his family. Cheryl replied that she did not know them. She was there because her pastor was doing the eulogy and that she came to hear him preach.

I was in search of a new church home and I thought to myself, what kind of preacher is this? Here is someone who took off of their day job, to come to a funeral of someone they did not know, just to hear the preacher preach! Instead of leaving the funeral home, I turned around and listened to the preacher. I had to see this for myself.

Never in my life have I heard a eulogy preached like that. I was completely spell-bound, and I knew that I was going to find this man's church. The name of the church, I found out later that day was Greater Love.

Now that I was in this prayer meeting, I knew that God was speaking directly to me.

Entering into the sunlight

Blessed are they which do hunger and thirst for righteousness: for they shall be filled.
Matthew 5: 6
NRSV Version

💟 Greater Love Christian Church
A life changing experience...

I walked in the door of the church and the pastor was already in the pulpit. As I was being escorted to my seat, Bishop Michael Barringer said, "You shall live and not die and declare the works of the Lord". I was stunned. How did he know what I was facing? He continued this sermon on healing, and I suspected that this was exactly where God wanted me to be.

I have gone to church most of my life. I have enjoyed the messages and I always prayed. But this experience was different. The energy that was in this church was intense. In my prior church experiences, I had encountered a lot of quasi Christians. You know the type that act like a Christian, talk like a Christian, and sometimes even walk like a Christian. I know this type of Christian because for so long, I was one of them.

I was able to quickly assess that the people in this church had a relationship with a real, living God. And even if the church body was not all the way there, I could tell that the pastor certainly was. This man could PREACH! And what was more amazing was how well he could TEACH. When I left that first service, I knew that I would return and worship there again. I did not know at that time; how pivotal this church would become in my life.

I do not think of myself as a church groupie or a preacher groupie. As Christians, we can sometimes become infatuated in our spiritual walk. We often romanticize and even idolize the church, its physical structure, and its leadership. But my experience in this church was undeniably positive. Sunday after Sunday, the messages of healing and restoration changed my outlook on life. I was being introduced to a real, living God. This God thing was infectious, and I could not get enough.

Those messages became my lifeline. It was as if the pastor was speaking directly to me, every Sunday. I left there each week empowered with the word of God.

Over time, I found myself going to church even if it meant that I had to walk. It was the first time that my soul was being fed at this level. My life had changed but the messages that I was receiving Sunday after Sunday were changing everything inside of me. My spiritual walk and my spiritual life completely changed.

There were so many sermons which had an impact on me. Two in particular stand out. The name of one sermon was called "The Place." I cannot recall the name of the other sermon but the content, I will never forget.

The sermon entitled "The Place" was relevant because the pastor spoke about reaching a marker in life where you have an encounter with God. This encounter with God is so extreme that it requires you to choose either to move closer to God in complete surrender or it is so overwhelming that you choose to retreat far from God. But it is a place that we all must encounter at some time in our lives as our Christian walk and purpose becomes clearer.

I was in that place. My outer circumstances appeared to be so dire and so hopeless. But my inner being was growing stronger in God's word. I was walking closer to God and surrendering to God's total will.

This sermon also spoke about transitioning out of your hurt and your shame and moving to "the place" where God wants you to be. Bishop Barringer said that when you cross over you can look back at the "tomb" of where and what you used be. The entire church was shouting.

There was another sermon that completely changed my direction and my understanding of what God had purposed for my life. This sermon was based on Roman's 8: 28-33.

28 And we know that in all things God works for the good of those who love him, who have been called according to his purpose.

29 For those God foreknew he also predestined to be conformed to the image of his Son, that he might be the firstborn among many brothers and sisters.

30 And those he predestined, he also called; those he called, he also justified; those he justified, he also glorified.

31 What, then, shall we say in response to these things? If God is for us, who can be against us?

32 He who did not spare his own Son, but gave him up for us all – how will he not also, along with him, graciously give us all things?

The pastor was speaking about our creation and our predestination. He said that we were created for the glorification of God. Before we were born, while we were still in our heavenly realm, God called us and asked if we would serve Him and we said, "Yes, Lord'. Then God proceeded to show us God's plans for our lives and we still said, "Yes, Lord." All of the peaks and all of the valleys were revealed. All of our test was shown to us and we told the Lord to send us and we would honor Him.

The pastor explained that God gives us free will. In the course of our human lives we forgot about the vision that God gave us. We sometimes forgot about God. But God never forgot us, and God never forgot about the plans for our lives.

The pastor went on to say that God knew that if we encountered adversity that He could count on us to withstand it. Because of what God put in each one of us, He knew the ones who could survive, no matter what.

This sermon really struck a chord with me. I knew that God was using me, but I did not know why. This sermon helped me realize that whatever I was going through, no matter how difficult, that God had specifically ordained it for my life. The "why" now became crystal clear.

It blew my mind to know that everything that I had experienced or that I ever will experience has been prearranged by God. This sermon gave me something tangible to grasp onto. My life and my experiences were for the glorification of God.

Ironically, I had spoken this same thing to Dr. Lavigne almost a year before I heard this sermon. Even though I did not fully understand the source of this truth, nevertheless, I understood it as truth when I spoke it.

Nothing in my life experience was news to God. I did not have to wait on God to work out my situation because He had already established the plans for my life. God was waiting on me to let God have total control. It was no longer about me and how was I going to get through. It was truly all about God. This sermon helped me to surrender all of my reasoning to the will of God and to move out of the way.

33 Who will bring any charge against those whom God has chosen? It is God who justifies.

I had been in surrender. I had an unwavering faith. I trusted God. But now I understood my true purpose. And nothing was going to keep me from it.

Hand polished and dried off by the best- -God himself

For I know the plans I have for you," declares the LORD, "plans to prosper you and not to harm you, plans to give you hope and a future."
Jeremiah 29:11
New International Version

Whenever you enter a car wash, you never really question the process. Whether you stay inside of the car or watch behind the glass as the car moves through, there is an excited anticipation of reaching the end.

At the time I began this journey, I had no idea that I would come to know God on such an intimate level. From the beginning, from the day I got the letter, from the moment that I came to my spiritual senses, I have lived in total trust of God. My faith has been admired by people hearing my story and I know that it has nothing to do with me.

God has allowed me to realize that my journey was purposed in order that I would know how to look to God no matter what the circumstance may bring. And God also purposed my journey so that people could see the radiant light of God within me.

As I have grown spiritually, I have come to understand that I am exactly where God wants me to be at each and every moment.

I can look back at each aspect of my journey through breast cancer and know that it was in fact orchestrated by God beginning with the castor oil that Neeka provided.

The bible tells us in Mark 6, verse 8 that Jesus commanded the disciples to take nothing for their journey, save a staff only, no scrip, no bread, no money in their purse.

I have come to understand that every tangible loss that I experienced during this time: my income, my house, my car, my possessions were ordained for the work that God has planned for me.

In the height of my illness I heard a song by Bishop Paul Morton, *"I'm Still Standing"* and it became my battle cry. The lyrics say that "I'm standing on the *word* that's in my heart."

Many people believe in God, but I have come to understand that there is a difference between believing in God and believing on the "word" of God.

Isaiah 55:11 tells us:

So is my word that goes out from my mouth: It will not return to me empty but will accomplish what I desire and achieve the purpose for which I sent it.

John 1:1 tells us that in the beginning was the Word, and the Word was with God, and the Word was God. Verses 1-5 go on to say,

In the beginning was the Word, and the Word was with God, and the Word was God. 2 He was with God in the beginning. 3 Through him all things were made; without him nothing was made that has been made. 4 In him was life, and that life was the light of all mankind. 5 The light shines in the darkness, and the darkness has not overcome it.

I have found that knowing and speaking God's word releases power in the spiritual realm that cannot be stopped. God's word is incapable of returning void.

I just recently came to the understanding that my walking was also ordained. There are two scriptures that come to mind. The first one is Luke 17:12-14. It tells of the story of the ten leapers and how Jesus healed them as they went.

The second scripture comes from St. John 5:8-9, in which Jesus was speaking to a disabled man lying by the pool of Bethesda.

8Then Jesus said to him, "Get up! Pick up your mat and walk." 9At once the man was cured; he picked up his mat and walked.

I literally walked into my healing.

I have come to understand that there is no way better than God's way. I began this journey with a desire to follow naturopathic medicine. My experience in Aruba allowed me to experience a hint of what was to come. I pursued a number of treatment options, some successful and some not so successful. I met several people along my path. But nothing can compare to God's healing plan.

The tumor that was in my breast is no more. The tumor in my lymph nodes is no more. My breast has completely closed, and it is covered with fresh new tissue. I have an indentation in my breast where the tumor once was, just like the "tomb" that Bishop Barringer had spoken about. I call it my *spiritual tattoo*. Whenever I have challenges or whenever I have doubt, I have a visible, tangible reminder that I was healed and touched by the hand of God.

I was speaking to Dr. Lavigne on my last visit and I told her how good I felt. She asked me if I had any pain and I told her that I did not have pain anywhere in my body. I said, "Dr. Lavigne, I don't even remember the cancer."

Yes, I know what I have been through, but it is no longer in the forethought of my mind. It is as if everything in my past never happened. God's healing is absolute.

In many ways the physician who gave me my death sentence was right. I did perhaps die but not in the way that she predicted. My fears died. My pain died. My hurts died. My will died. My open breast looked like an impossible situation. My depleted finances looked like an impossible situation. But the God I serve specializes in fixing and curing the impossible.

I have a new resurrected life in God.

I have recently answered a call to the ministry, and I cannot wait to see where God is taking me. My spiritual journey through breast cancer has prepared me for just about anything.

I have come to know that it was only in my broken places that I learned to keep my eye solely on God. It was only in my nothingness that I finally found a love; a fellowship; and a communion without compare.

I am moved by the knowledge that I found in Isaiah 43:

> *"Do not fear, for I have redeemed you;*
> *   I have summoned you by name; you are mine.*
> *2 When you pass through the waters,*
> *   I will be with you;*
> *and when you pass through the rivers,*
> *   they will not sweep over you.*
> *When you walk through the fire,*
> *   you will not be burned;*
> *   the flames will not set you ablaze.*
> *3 For I am the Lord your God,*
> *   the Holy One of Israel, your Savior;*
> *I give Egypt for your ransom,*
> *   Cush and Seba in your stead.*
> *4 Since you are precious and honored in my sight,*
> *   and because I love you,*
> *I will give people in exchange for you,*
> *   nations in exchange for your life.*

5 *Do not be afraid, for I am with you;*
   I will bring your children from the east
   and gather you from the west.
6 *I will say to the north, 'Give them up!'*
   and to the south, 'Do not hold them back.'
Bring my sons from afar
   and my daughters from the ends of the earth –
7 *everyone who is called by my name,*
   whom I created for my glory,
   whom I formed and made."
8 *Lead out those who have eyes but are blind,*
   who have ears but are deaf.
9 *All the nations gather together*
   and the peoples assemble.
Which of their gods foretold this
   and proclaimed to us the former things?
Let them bring in their witnesses to prove they
were right,
   so that others may hear and say, "It is true."
10 *"You are my witnesses," declares the Lord,*
   "and my servant whom I have chosen,
so that you may know and believe me
   and understand that I am he.
Before me no god was formed,
   nor will there be one after me.

I rejoice in knowing that God knows me by
name.

SPECIAL NOTE

The treatment that I received as outlined in this book was unique to my journey. In following your journey, the outcome might be much different. I am sharing my story to give you hope in the unlimited abilities of God, through His son, Jesus Christ. I respect traditional medicine and I respect naturopathic options. It is my hope that through my story, both communities will look differently at one another.

I believe that it is my fundamental right to choose my own healthcare and my own treatment options. But within our current health system, this right is severely impaired. Because of the limitations placed on naturopathic practitioners, some of the best treatment options are ignored. I do advocate for some degree of regulations because it will eliminate a few individuals who engage in quackery. I have found in most instances, if a true practitioner cannot help you, they will not hurt you.

Prior to my diagnosis, I never questioned anything that a doctor told me. Please understand that I have tremendous respect for medical doctors. But I have learned through this experience, to seek guidance from a number of different sources.

In many ways, I have become a student of natural remedies. I have learned a great deal about both herbs and medicine; and the impact that they have on the body. As a personal practice, I seek

101

natural options first. I use traditional medicine only as a last resort.

I have learned that cancer attacks the body on a cellular level. Each one of us is uniquely made and my cellular composition is not like anyone else. The point that I am making is cancer treatment has to become more individualized. No two people will have the exact same reactions or the exact same outcome.

The core biopsy revealed that I was both an estrogen and a progesterone receptor. The cancer in my breast is hormonally driven. The chemo combination that I was scheduled to receive was deemed standard cancer treatment for my staging. This combination would have never effectively treated me because it did not address the hormonal issue that was driving the cancer.

My breast first opened in July 2005 and it continued to open until September 2006. From September 2006 until May 2007, the tumor was at a standstill. It neither grew nor did it shrink. From June 2007 to February 2008, the tumor grew beyond description.

The first significant shrinkage that I experienced since Aruba occurred after I had taken the Chinese herbs in February 2008. I then started the Tamoxifen in April 2008. My breast began closing in August 2008, although I still had a large hole. By mid-2009, my breast was beginning to be covered with a scab. By January 2010, the scab was gone, and fresh new skin appeared. By May 2010, only the calcified tumor remained. On June 1, 2010, all of my blood work came back clear.

Whatever medical path that you that you follow, make sure that you align yourself with professional practitioners that you are comfortable with. Acting alone because you read about a new cure on the internet is definitely not the path to follow. Every person that I consulted was well versed in his or her perspective field. I did a lot of research. I asked a lot of questions.

Most importantly, never underestimate the power of prayer and the power of divine guidance. God is faithful. Allow God to order your steps and direct your path.

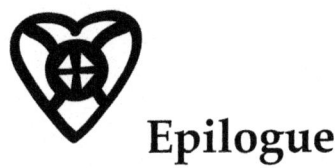 Epilogue

It has been ten years since I initially wrote the front part of this book. So much has happened in my life over these past ten years. I pursued advanced theological training at Howard University School of Divinity and received a Master of Divinity Degree in May 2014.

Many of the people who were a part of my spiritual journey are no longer here. Over the years, I have lost my beloved grandmother at the age of 99 years old. I lost my father; Alan Price; and my dear friend Carmen. I am so grateful that they graced my presence. I am a much better person for the imprint that they left on my life.

I am working in ministry full time and I am keenly aware that my ministry is rooted in both story and voice. I am a firm believer in the power of story.

Often, when we encounter difficulties, we make an unfortunate assumption that a particular situation happens uniquely to us. Sometimes in our need for both privacy and understanding, we hide our stories, or we become ashamed about our stories without realizing that our difficulties or adversity is never really about us: even if it impacts us personally.

Our experiences and our stories are for the encouragement and uplifting of others who perhaps, unaware, are facing a similar situation. It is in the sharing of our own unique story that we are able to connect with others, to understand others, and most importantly, to have empathy for another human being. The sharing of our story moves it from one of personal ownership to one of communal ownership, thus uniting us in our human journey.

In writing this book, I realized early on that my story would help another cancers survivor along their journey. When I gave this book a title, I understood that I was on a spiritual journey. However, I never thought that I would tell this story again as a cancer patient. But here I find myself confronting breast cancer once again. It is confirmation that my spiritual journey continues. I am sure that it is rare for the words honor and cancer to appear together, but I do somehow count it an honor to bring this story to you. I am constantly reminded of the faithfulness of God. I am a living testament that God is ever present, ever healing.

I began to notice some problems with my breast in the spring of 2015. I was in denial on some levels because I did not feel like dealing with the possibility of breast cancer again. By October 2015, I was undeniably back in a similar space unconscionable pain. I had the type of moaning and tear-filled pain that only advance cancer can bring. Advance cancer is a very, very painful experience. Even with medication, it is very difficult to escape the pain. I cannot adequately describe the pain; there are no words that can adequately explain the excessive amount of pain that cancer can bring.

Before Labor Day, I had planned a trip back to Cincinnati to see my oncologist. If this was cancer again, I decided that is where I would start. They were familiar with my history and my belief system. So, I decided that I would start there. However, each time I would attempt to make travel arrangements, I would encounter a distraction. There appeared to be some emergency or crisis every day.

By early October, I did not care what other crisis was on the table, I had to find the time to get back to Cincinnati. I finally made the trip on a Thursday. My girlfriend from college picked me up and did not say a negative word. However, the look on her face gave me an indicator of her concern.

I had lost a whole lot of weight since we had last seen one another. I mean a lot of weight. I was aware of the weight loss because my clothes no longer fit. But I was not aware of how I look through the eyes of someone else. My girlfriend has always been cool; it is a Mid-West trademark. But she later expressed her concern and was praying that I would get better soon. I told her that I did not know if I had any fight left in me. I had fought so long, through so many things; I just did not know if there was any more fight left.

We left early the next morning and she dropped me off at the doctor. I slept when I reached her home the day before. The pain was surreal, so I tried to remain quiet and just endure.

I arrived at the doctor's office with no scheduled appointment. I had been making appointment after appointment, but I could never make the trip. The last time I talked to the doctor's scheduler she said just show up whenever and we will fit you in. When I got to the window, I introduced myself. At long last we finally meet. I explain that I did not have an appointment and that she had told me over the phone that they would fit me in. She looked at me and said, "Oh no, you do have a scheduled appointment. We have you scheduled at ten o'clock this morning." Okay, I am thinking, "God, I see you." Somehow in all of our conversations, she inadvertently scheduled me for that day and for that particular time. It was confirmation that God was still orchestrating, arranging and coordinating the affairs in my life.

I met with the oncologist and he remembered my case. Once again, my breast was open and bleeding. We talked about options and he made an herbal compound for me to take. He also suggested that I begin a regime of an oral chemotherapy called Letrozole. Because I have been successful with Tamoxifen in the past, he felt like this new chemotherapy would work as well. He explained that the type of cancer in my body is hormonally driven. I would always have to be concerned about my hormone levels for the rest of my life. He explained that as long as I lived, the body would produce hormones. My goal is effective management of the hormones.

He suggested that I stay in the area for overall effective treatment. I explained that I no longer lived in Ohio and that my insurance was in another state. I promised to keep in touch and let him know how I was doing. With herbs and prescription in hand, I traveled to Dayton to see my family. Another girlfriend picked me up and I ended up spending the weekend at her house.

My experience with active advanced cancer has been one of extreme pain. At this point it was difficult to sleep during the night. Every time I would lie down, the pain in my breast would beat like a very loud and violently banging drum. The only way that I could sleep was to sit up flat against the wall. I would prop pillows up on both sides to make sure that I would not lie down. On this weekend visit to my girlfriend, she had a chaise lounge and I stayed on that lounge all of the time. It marked the second time in a while that I had slept without being awakened by the pain.

I returned to the Washington, DC area and I noticed that the pain had subsided just a little. I was taking the herbal compound daily. I also began to take the oral chemo. I then contacted my local healthcare provider and set up an appointment. This was at the end of October and I was to see a new primary care physician on November 3, 2015. I was enthusiastic in the most sarcastic way. The last thing on my agenda was to confront another bout with cancer. On top of that, I really did not feel like starting over with new doctors; explaining my history; being judged; and slightly mistreated as I had experienced in the past. I just wanted it to all go away. I did not want to be bothered.

The idea of this being a spiritual journey was nowhere in my thought process. I was lamenting to my niece Rhea about how disinterested I was in going to the doctor the next day. I was telling her that I did not feel like going through this again. It was a basic evening of lamenting and complaining. My niece reminded me that I had a responsibility to follow-through (which I knew, but the complaining which I never do, felt right at the moment).

I went to sleep that Monday night and there was a peace that came over me. When I woke up the next day, it was as if none of the lamenting and complaining matter. I told my niece that I was looking forward to going to the doctor. I thought that I had my fight back. It was as if God had spoken to me through the night, "Let's go, you CAN get through this."

I arrived at my doctor's office early Tuesday morning. I participate in a managed health plan, so I understood that this was the first doctor that I was going to see. I had to go through her to get an appointment with the oncologist. In my mind, I did not want to spend a lot of time here because I knew that it was an oncological issue. I was hoping for a short visit and then I could go on to the next step.

This particular doctor is an African American woman with a very quiet spirit. She is unassuming and at first, I was not sure that she was the physician assigned to my case. She introduced herself and then we relocated to another office. I gave my full history as well as the report from my doctor in Cincinnati. She listened tentatively and asked routine questions. Her major concern was the stroke level blood pressure. I explained my history and the level of stress that I constantly endure. She made it clear that it was an issue that would be addressed.

We spent at least an hour together gathering history and perhaps adjusting to our new relationship. As long as I was under this health plan, I would see this physician for every consultation and referral that I needed. She was thorough and took her time. She excused herself and at the end of the visit, she said, "I like to leave my patients with three things when they leave." I honestly do not remember the first two things she said but I will never forget the last thing she wanted to leave--prayer. I almost jumped out of my chair! (She said she would like to leave me with PRAYER?) I could not believe my ears, but I give thanks on this day and forevermore that this woman of faith is my physician. In my opinion, there is no more intimate experience than prayer. And to begin this journey for the second time with a faith-filled physician was simply mind-blowing.

.

We begin to prayer together: two strangers. She prayed for my healing and that God would continually be glorified in my experience. I prayed and gave thanks that God saw fit to send me to a woman of faith to begin my healing journey. I was so moved by her unashamedly love for God. I will always be grateful for that moment.

The doctor scheduled me to see an oncologist. I was not sure what to expect. After having met my primary care physician, I was prepared for just about anything. I was no longer lamenting so I arrived early, looking forward to getting on the other side of this experience.

The oncologist entered the room. He confirmed that I was in fact the correct patient and then he spoke. "I want to tell you what an honor it is to meet you," extending his hand. "You are a living miracle, and I am so honored to meet you today. You have been dealing with cancer over the past twelve years and to still be alive and in good health, you are a miracle."

I felt relaxed in his presence. We discussed treatment options and I shared with him about my commitment to naturopathic options. He told me that he would support whatever course of treatment that I decided to follow. He recommended an additional chemotherapy treatment, a new "miracle" drug which was recently approved by the FDA. He believed that the combination of these two drugs would put me in remission very quickly. With every medical decision that I have made, I have always conducted research and I pray. Then only and only then do I make a decision about my healthcare. It is always done in spiritual consultation. I told the oncologist that I would research the other drug: that I would pray and seek guidance; and then I would let him know of my decision.

The second chemotherapy that the oncologist suggested had a few side effects would impact my blood count and it would require frequent blood transfusions. I prayed for guidance and ultimately decided against the second chemotherapy.

I began a new battery of tests to see where I was with my staging. When the PET Scan results came back, it was determined that it was again at Stage VI localized in the left breast. I counted it as a blessing because I did not have to worry about other organs. But I later found out that the PET Scan showed that the cancer had metastasized in the lymph node and in the bone. But at the time, sharing with me that the cancer was localized put a different focus on my fight. I was diagnosed with Stage IV metastasis breast cancer. I understood metastasis in terms of recurring but not in terms of spreading. Had I known it was outside of the breast, I am not sure that I would have had the strength to fight. I took on the been-there-done attitude and went on with my life.

I was constantly at the doctor's office for testing, evaluation, and results. I had several back to-back visits from November through February. What I love about my healthcare provider is that everything is digital. As soon as the test results are back, they are posted immediately. You have the opportunity to know at all times the status of your health. There are certain results, however, that are not posted such as the PET Scan. You must see the doctor for the results.

By the beginning of January, my breast was starting to close again and the pain was almost nonexistent. I was celebrating my progress, giving thanks for each good report. But by March things were changing in my body.

I was constantly cold--freezing cold. I could not be in the house without being under a blanket. I would get so cold that I would shiver and shake. It would take hours before I would feel any warmth.

Other changes begin to take place as well. I was losing weight rapidly. Week after week I was losing five, seven, eight pounds. The weight just continued to drop. As a full-figured woman mostly all of my life, the goal is to be less than 200 pounds; and only people who are over 200 pounds know what I am talking about. It is everyone's goal to get below 200 pounds even if the scales read 199.9 pounds. It is less than 200 pounds no matter how you look at it. In my case, the first time the scales reached below 200 pounds, I did not even celebrate because I knew that I was sick. As the weight continued to drop, I told the Lord that I was grateful for how fabulous I looked but I did not want to be fabulous and dead at the same time.

The weight loss was a major concern for me. It was an indicator that major changes were occurring in my body. One of the last changes that took place was my inability to eat. Aha, that could explain the weight loss but, in my mind, I felt like I was eating. I had a full appetite. I still had a taste for food. I just could not eat very much of it. I was still walking two to three miles every day so maybe that is why the weight kept dropping off. I communicated my concern to my oncologist because

I knew that I was not getting enough caloric intake to support the amount of medication that I was taking. I still had a desire and taste for food, but I could only eat very small portion. Oh Lord, please do not tell me that my fifty-plus years love affair with food was ending. I was baffled.

I went to see my oncologist in May 2016. By this time, my breast is completely closed, and new pink skin was on the horizon. Hallelujah! I could not honestly remember the pain. Glory to God! It had been months since I had taken a Tylenol. I knew that healing was taking place in my body. I did not have a true worry, but I was concerned about the rapid weight loss.

My oncologist was excited about my progress. He stated that he wanted to be responsible and have a new battery of test done. He ordered blood work and a new PET Scan. He also suggested that we look at the brain to rule out any further spreading. I heard him as it relates to spreading so I agreed to ruling out any spreading. At the time I was unaware of the initial diagnosis which did indicate that the cancer was in the lymph node and in the bone, but my oncologist was aware. I found out on this day in May that the first report identified the cancer in all three locations: the breast, lymph node; and bone: pretty much everywhere. I was floored by the report, but I was not afraid. I just wanted to know why that had not been shared with me originally.

Now I had a better understanding about the weight loss and the loss of appetite. I was fighting a bigger battle than I thought. I was more than ever trusting God for a better outcome.

I was scheduled to see a Nephrologist regarding my uncontrollable hypertension. He had some concerns as well about the functioning of my kidneys. According to the test results, the kidneys were in terrible shape. He spoke to me about a low sodium diet and then he looked on the screen.

He said, "It looks like the cancer is fairly aggressive, so we won't spend a lot of time with your diet. The main thing that I want you to do is to experience joy and to be happy." Then he continued; if the cancer continues to be aggressive, then there will be no need to worry about the kidneys. Just work on finding some joy in your life."

I really did not know what to say. I was at a loss for words. I had just had my new PET Scan a few days before this visit. Maybe my oncologist had not had a chance to let me know how bad things had become. On my last visit with my oncologist, I learned about the spreading but because my breast had closed and I was not in any pain, I knew that some type of healing had taken place. All I could think was what in the world is going on.

I met the Nephrologist on the first Tuesday in June. I had to go to Ohio to my uncle's funeral. I did not want to carry the burden of my medical news with me, so I put it out of my mind until I returned. I told a friend of mine who was in constant prayer with me that I had to have a resolve on some things from my doctor. I did not tell her what was said to me, only that I would confront it upon my return.

Monday could not arrive soon enough. If I was really terminally, I wanted all of the details: no holding back. I contacted my oncologist via email because I wanted to know what the PET Scan results indicated. I got a reply immediately from Hematology stating that only my oncologist could speak to me. I was slightly frustrated because I do not know how Hematology got in the conversation. I reasoned that it must be pretty serious, so I waited patiently for his reply.

About three hours later, I get a reply as follows:

"The PET CT scan shows abnormal activity only in your primary tumor and no longer in any metastases, and the tumor activity has also decreased. Based on this good report, no need for a brain MRI now."

Even with the exciting news, I still did not feel good. I was sluggish and overall weak. I did not have the will or the strength for my daily walk even though I made attempts often. One week in July I was so sick that I did not return any phone calls. I stayed in bed and rested. I just felt sick.

I happened to go to the store, and I ran into a friend. The month before, he had given me his research to review. I had not looked at it. I had not felt like it and I LOVE research. When I got home that night, I reviewed and edited his materials.

I called him early the next morning and told him that I wanted to meet him to return his research. I was going to meet him early in the day, but I did not feel well so it took several hours for me to gather the strength to meet him. When we finally met, the very first thing I said to him was how sick I felt. I told him, "I wanted to make sure that I gave you your thumb drive back in the event that I die. My family would not know what it means to you and you could lose your research." I knew that I was that kind of sick. After our meeting I decided to go to bed until I could get a handle on my health.

The next day was Sunday and I knew that I was not going anywhere. I was determined to recover, and I knew that rest would take care of everything. I stayed in bed all day. I had no energy and I had been nauseated for months.

I woke up the next morning very nauseous. I realized that I had not eaten since Saturday. I knew that I had to eat but the nausea would allow me to eat. I got up to go get breakfast and I started to walk. I went about 500 feet and almost collapsed. My heart was racing, and I could barely breathe. I have never experienced shortness of breath. What is this? What is going on?

I sat for about twenty minutes and I started to ask the maintenance man on the property to give me a ride back to my apartment. But there was a Godly nudge pressing me to keep going. I had neither strength nor energy, but I got up and moved. I made it about another 500 feet, and I knew that I was going to collapse. I have never fainted before. I have felt like I wanted to faint, but I have never actually fainted. But I knew it was a matter of seconds before I hit the ground.

Only two thoughts were going on in my mind, one, Lord do not let me hit my head on this sidewalk and two, help me to call 911 so that my family can find me. I did not want to be a Jane Doe who had died on the sidewalk. I had no expectation of living and I did not have one ounce of fight left in me. It was truly a surrender moment. If it was my last day on earth, I was at total peace.

I managed to get my phone out of my purse, and I dialed 911. I identified myself and my location and I passed out. I was unaware that the 911 operator was trying to reach me. When I came to, my phone was buzzing. I managed to find the phone. I told the operator that I could not talk, and he told me not to talk but I had to stay on the line until EMS arrived. In the faint background, I could hear the siren. It felt like an eternity but within a few minutes, they had arrived.

I explained that I was a cancer patient and I just felt weak. They transported me to the hospital, and I knew that I would be there for a while. I soon learned that I was anemic, and all of the symptoms lined up under anemia. It created a domino effect. The anemia caused the nausea; the nausea caused the gastritis; the gastritis cause dehydration. I have never been so sick in my entire life. One of my bragging points is that I never experienced any side effects from cancer. I know excruciating pain, but I have never known near death illness: the kind that you do not even care if you live or die. I have never known that kind of sickness.

I give thanks for that Godly nudge to press on. Had I been able to return home, I more than likely would not be here. My blood count was so low. I was given a blood transfusion; I.V.'s; and anti-nausea medication. After several days, I was finally discharged from the hospital.

I left the hospital feeling better but not great. I was still weak and very nauseous. The nurse explained that I was stable, but I was going to feel "crappy" for a while. In my mind, a while was a few more days. It ended up taking seven more weeks before I saw a glimpse of my former self.

I have continued to battle cancer even after this second bout. I am gaining strength daily and I have come to understand the importance of my life. My cancer numbers continue to trend low! I am of the belief that God has spared me once again to tell the story and to serve as a reminder that God still performs miracles, daily.

We often assign every negative situation as an attack of the enemy. We give so much credit for our circumstances as being outside the realm or will of God. My story reminds one that God never takes his hands, eyes, or love away from our lives. God is ever present, even if we cannot feel him. God is constantly arranging, coordinating and directing the course of our lives. Our charge is to trust God even when it defies logic.

In our surrendered lives, God allows us to experience things that are sometimes unpleasant and hurtful, but it will always serve as propeller rather than a hindrance. The experience will move one to greater heights and to a greater faith. I know because the journey through breast cancer brought me to a relationship with a living God. Cancer was the catalyst that appeared to be evil but in reality, it became my good. This journey brought me to ministry and to share the good news that God never leaves us nor forsakes us. God is with us always. God simply is.

ACKNOWLEDGEMENT

I am indebted to a number of people who have supported me and my son during this journey. It would be impossible to list everyone. There are so many people who prayed for me; stood in the gap with me; provided resources to me; and cheered me every step of the way. You know who you are, and I know who you are. Your love is forever written on my heart. For every prayer and petition sent on my behalf, I thank you. For every ounce of compassion given to me, I thank you.

If you or your organization would like to host a book signing; order books; or if you would like to host me as a speaker, please contact me at info@jspublishing.me.

May God's abundant blessings continue to spring forth in your lives. To God be the Glory for the great things that God has done!

Printed in Great Britain
by Amazon

66356765R00081